# Pilates For Seniors Over 50

The ultimate guide on easy-to-follow low impact home exercises for enhancing balance, stability and posture

**Gano Picard**

# Table of content

# Introduction

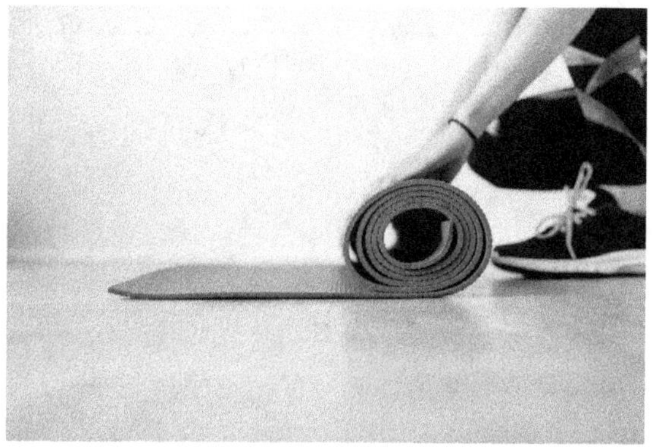

Pilates, a holistic exercise method developed by Joseph Pilates in the early 20th century, has gained widespread recognition for its transformative effects on physical fitness and overall well-being. In recent years, the focus on adapting Pilates for seniors has become increasingly prominent, recognizing the unique needs and health considerations of the aging population. This introduction aims to provide an insightful overview of Pilates for seniors and delve into the manifold benefits it offers to older adults.

# Overview

As individuals age, maintaining a healthy and active lifestyle becomes paramount for preserving mobility, flexibility, and overall vitality. Pilates, with its emphasis on controlled movements, breath awareness, and core strength, proves to be an ideal exercise form for seniors seeking to enhance their physical health and quality of life.

Pilates for seniors involves a tailored approach that takes into account the specific challenges and considerations associated with aging bodies. Unlike high-impact exercises, Pilates is gentle on the joints, making it accessible for individuals with varying degrees of mobility and fitness levels. The exercises can be easily modified to accommodate specific needs, ensuring a safe and effective workout for seniors.

One of the key principles of Pilates, core strength, holds particular significance for seniors. A strong core contributes to improved balance and stability, crucial elements for preventing falls and maintaining independence. The focus on controlled movements in Pilates helps seniors develop better body awareness, promoting a sense of balance and coordination that is invaluable for everyday activities.

Moreover, Pilates for seniors encompasses a holistic approach, addressing not only physical but also mental well-being. The mindful nature of Pilates exercises encourages a deeper connection between the body and the mind, fostering mental clarity and reducing stress – factors that are especially pertinent for seniors facing the challenges of aging.

## Benefits of Pilates for Older Adults:

1. Improved Core Strength and Stability:
   Pilates places a strong emphasis on the core muscles, including the abdominals, back, and pelvic floor. For seniors, this translates to enhanced core strength, providing stability and support for daily activities, such as standing, walking, and bending.

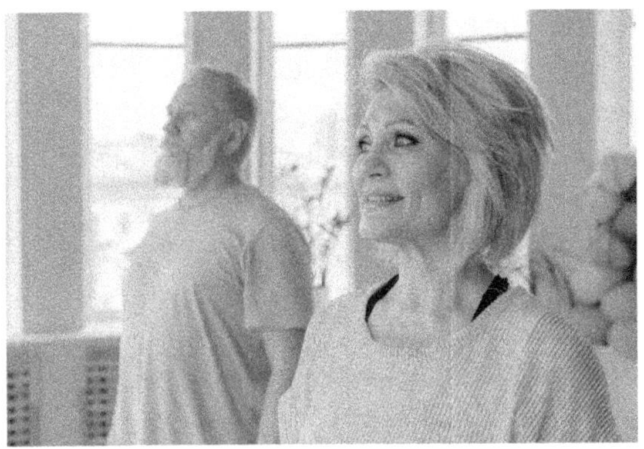

2. Enhanced Flexibility and Joint Mobility:
Aging often brings a decrease in flexibility and joint mobility. Pilates counteracts these effects through a range of gentle stretches and movements, promoting flexibility and maintaining a full range of motion in the joints.

3. Balance and Coordination Enhancement:
The emphasis on controlled movements in Pilates contributes to improved balance and coordination. This is particularly beneficial for seniors who may experience challenges in these areas, reducing the risk of falls and injuries.

4. Stress Reduction and Mindfulness:

Pilates integrates breath awareness and mindfulness into its practice, providing seniors with a therapeutic outlet for stress reduction. Engaging in mindful movement not only improves physical health but also contributes to mental well-being.

5. Joint-Friendly Exercise:

Many seniors deal with joint issues, such as arthritis or stiffness. Pilates offers a low-impact alternative that is gentle on the joints, making it accessible for those with various physical conditions.

6. Posture Improvement:

As the body ages, maintaining good posture becomes crucial for spinal health. Pilates encourages proper alignment and awareness of body posture, aiding in the prevention of issues related to poor alignment, such as back pain.

7. Adaptable to Individual Needs:

Pilates is inherently adaptable, allowing instructors to tailor exercises to suit individual needs and limitations. Whether a senior is a beginner or more advanced, Pilates can be modified to accommodate their unique abilities and challenges.

In conclusion, Pilates embodies a holistic approach to fitness and well-being, addressing the physical, mental, and emotional aspects of health.

# Chapter 1

# Getting Started with Pilates for Seniors

Pilates, a renowned exercise system developed by Joseph Pilates, has gained popularity for its holistic approach to physical fitness and well-being. Specifically tailored for seniors, Pilates offers a gentle yet effective means of enhancing strength, flexibility, and overall vitality. In this section, we will delve into the essential aspects of getting started with Pilates for seniors, covering preparation, safety considerations, and the appropriate equipment and attire.

## Preparing for Pilates

Embarking on a Pilates journey requires thoughtful preparation to ensure a safe and enjoyable experience. Before diving into the exercises, seniors should consider the following key aspects:

# 1. Health Assessment

Prior to starting any exercise program, it is crucial for seniors to undergo a health assessment. Consulting with a healthcare professional or a qualified fitness instructor can help identify any pre-existing health conditions or physical limitations that may require modifications to the Pilates routine.

# 2. Goal Setting

Establishing clear fitness goals is an integral part of preparation. Whether aiming to improve flexibility, build core strength, or enhance overall well-being, seniors should define their objectives to tailor their Pilates practice accordingly.

# 3. Mental Preparation

Pilates is not just a physical exercise but also involves mental focus and mindfulness. Seniors should approach Pilates with a positive mindset, embracing the mind-body connection that is central to the practice.

4. Consistency

Consistency is key to reaping the benefits of Pilates. Seniors should commit to a regular practice schedule, starting with manageable durations and gradually progressing as their comfort and strength increase.

## Safety Considerations

Safety is paramount, especially when engaging in physical activities, and Pilates is no exception. Seniors should be mindful of the following safety considerations:

1. Proper Form and Technique

Emphasizing proper form and technique is crucial to prevent injuries and maximize the effectiveness of Pilates exercises. Seniors should start with foundational movements, focusing on mastering each before progressing to more advanced exercises.

## 2. Avoiding Overexertion

While Pilates is a low-impact exercise, seniors should be cautious not to overexert themselves. Gradual progression is key, allowing the body to adapt and reduce the risk of strains or injuries.

## 3. Clear Communication

Open communication with instructors or workout partners is essential. Seniors should feel comfortable expressing any discomfort or concerns during their Pilates sessions to ensure that modifications can be made when necessary.

## 4. Breathing Awareness

Pilates places a strong emphasis on coordinated breathing with movement. Seniors should pay attention to their breath, inhaling and exhaling at the appropriate times, which not only enhances the effectiveness of the exercises but also promotes relaxation.


## Equipment and Attire


Selecting the right equipment and attire enhances the Pilates experience, providing comfort and support throughout the practice:


1. Mat
A non-slip, comfortable mat is a fundamental requirement for Pilates. It provides a cushioned surface for floor exercises, ensuring seniors can perform movements with stability and ease.

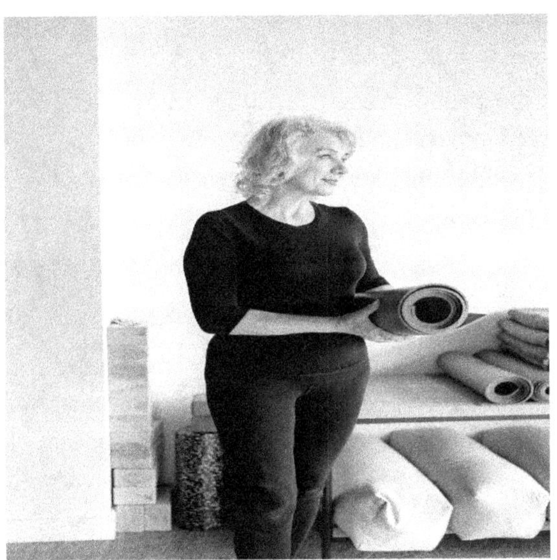

## 2. Props

While not mandatory, props such as resistance bands, stability balls, and Pilates rings can add variety and intensity to workouts. Seniors can gradually incorporate these props as they become more familiar with the basic Pilates exercises.

## 3. Comfortable Clothing

Wearing breathable, stretchable clothing allows for unrestricted movement during Pilates sessions. Opt for comfortable attire that does not constrict their range of motion.

## 4. Footwear

Pilates is typically performed barefoot or in socks to promote better grip and sensory feedback. However, if you have a specific foot condition you may choose supportive footwear with the approval of your healthcare provider.

By following these guidelines, you can embark on your Pilates journey with confidence, knowing that you  are setting yourself up for a fulfilling and rewarding experience.

# Chapter 2

# Warm-up Exercises

Warm-up exercises are an essential component of any Pilates routine, particularly for seniors. They help to prepare the body for movement, increase circulation, and reduce the risk of injury. In this section, we will explore three key aspects of warm-up exercises in Pilates: gentle joint movements, breathing techniques, and mobility exercises.

## Gentle Joint Movements

Gentle joint movements are a vital part of warming up the body before engaging in more strenuous activity. It is essential to start slowly and gently to avoid strain or injury. Here are some gentle joint movements that can be incorporated into a Pilates warm-up routine:

1. Neck Rolls: Slowly and gently roll the neck in a circular motion, first clockwise and then counterclockwise, to release tension and increase flexibility in the neck and shoulders.

2. Shoulder Rolls: Roll the shoulders forward and backward in a circular motion, gradually increasing the range of motion with each repetition. This helps to loosen up the shoulder joints and improve mobility.

3. Wrist Circles: Rotate the wrists in circular motions, first clockwise and then counterclockwise, to warm up the wrists and hands. This is especially beneficial for seniors who spend a lot of time typing or performing repetitive hand movements.

4. Ankle Circles: Sit or stand with feet flat on the ground and gently rotate the ankles in circular motions, first clockwise and then counterclockwise. This helps to improve mobility in the ankles and feet, reducing the risk of falls and injuries.

5. Hip Circles: Stand with feet hip-width apart and gently rotate the hips in circular motions, first clockwise and then counterclockwise. This helps to loosen up the hip joints and improve range of motion.

## Breathing Techniques

Breathing techniques are an integral part of Pilates, helping to promote relaxation, increase oxygen flow to the muscles, and enhance the mind-body connection. Focusing on proper breathing can also help to alleviate stress and anxiety. Here are some breathing techniques that can be incorporated into a Pilates warm-up routine:

1. Diaphragmatic Breathing:

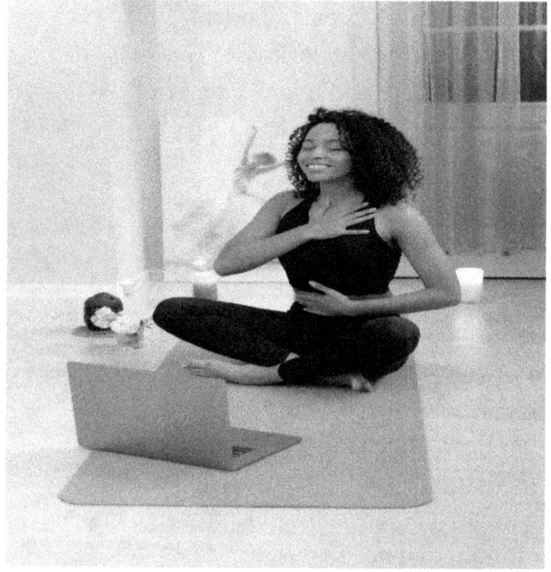

Sit or lie down comfortably and place one hand on the chest and the other on the abdomen. Inhale deeply through the nose, allowing the abdomen to expand fully, and then exhale slowly through the mouth, drawing the navel toward the spine. Repeat this deep breathing pattern several times, focusing on the sensation of the breath filling the lungs and belly.

2. Rib Cage Expansion: Sit or stand with arms by the sides and inhale deeply, expanding the rib cage laterally. Exhale slowly, drawing the ribs back together. This helps to improve thoracic mobility and increase lung capacity.

3. Segmental Breathing: Lie on the back with knees bent and feet flat on the floor. Place hands on the rib cage and inhale deeply, focusing on expanding one segment of the rib cage at a time, starting from the lower ribs and moving upward. Exhale slowly, releasing the breath from the upper ribs down to the lower ribs. This helps to increase awareness of the breath and improve breathing efficiency.

4. Breath with Movement: Coordinate breath with movement during warm-up exercises, inhaling to prepare for a movement and exhaling to execute the movement. This helps to synchronize breath and movement, promoting a fluid and controlled motion.

# Mobility Exercises

Mobility exercises are designed to increase range of motion and flexibility in the joints and muscles, helping seniors to maintain functional movement and prevent stiffness and pain. Here are some mobility exercises that can be incorporated into a Pilates warm-up routine:

## A. Cat-Cow Stretch:

The Cat-Cow Stretch is a simple yet effective yoga pose that helps to improve spinal flexibility and mobility. Here are the steps to perform the Cat-Cow Stretch:

1. Start on your hands and knees in a tabletop position. Your wrists should be directly under your shoulders, and your knees should be hip-width apart, directly under your hips. Ensure that your spine is in a neutral position, with your back flat and your neck in line with your spine.

2. As you inhale, begin the Cow position by arching your back and dropping your belly towards the floor. Lift your chest and gaze upward, allowing your tailbone to lift slightly towards the ceiling. This is the Cow position, and it should create a gentle stretch along the front of your torso.

3. As you exhale, transition into the Cat position by rounding your spine towards the ceiling, tucking your chin towards your chest, and drawing your belly button towards your spine. Feel a stretch along your upper back as you press firmly into the ground with your hands and knees. This is the Cat position.

4. Continue to flow between the Cat and Cow positions, moving with your breath. Inhale as you arch into Cow, and exhale as you round into Cat. Move slowly and mindfully, allowing your breath to guide your movements.

5. Repeat the Cat-Cow Stretch for several rounds, moving smoothly and fluidly with your breath. Pay attention to any areas of tension or tightness in your

spine, and focus on releasing and relaxing those areas with each repetition.

6. You can vary the movement by exploring different ranges of motion and adding gentle movements, such as circling the hips or swaying from side to side. Listen to your body and adjust the stretch as needed to suit your comfort level.

7. After completing several rounds of the Cat-Cow Stretch, return to a neutral tabletop position and take a moment to notice how your spine feels. You may notice increased flexibility and mobility, as well as a sense of relaxation and openness in your back.

8. To come out of the stretch, slowly transition into a seated or standing position, taking care to move mindfully and avoid any sudden movements.

## B. Seated Spinal Stretch:

The seated spine stretch is a fundamental Pilates exercise that targets the muscles of the spine, promoting flexibility and mobility.

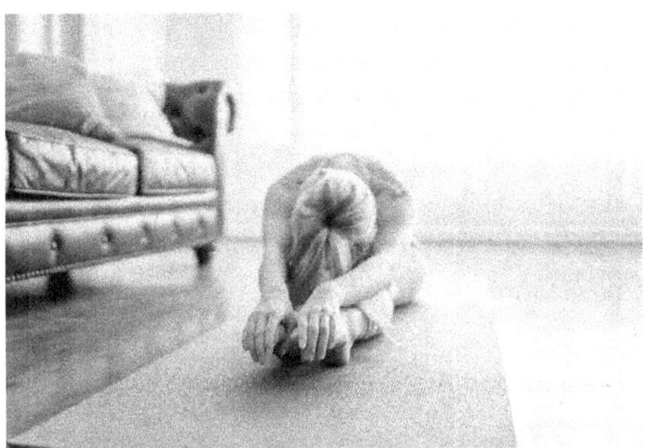

Here are the steps to perform the seated spine stretch:

1. Starting Position:
   - Sit tall on a mat or chair with your legs extended straight in front of you.
   - Ensure your feet are hip-width apart and flexed, with your toes pointing toward the ceiling.
   - Place your hands by your sides, resting on the mat or chair for support.

2. Inhale Preparation:
   - Inhale deeply through your nose, lengthening your spine and sitting up tall.

3. Exhale Forward Bend:
   - Exhale slowly as you initiate the movement by engaging your abdominal muscles.
   - Begin to articulate your spine forward, leading with your chest and keeping your shoulders relaxed.
   - Imagine reaching your crown towards your toes as you fold forward from your hips.
   - Keep your spine long and avoid rounding your back excessively.
   - Continue to exhale as you reach your hands towards your feet or shins, maintaining a gentle stretch through your spine.

4. Inhale Return to Start:
   - Inhale deeply as you reverse the movement, slowly stacking your spine back up to the starting position.
   - Initiate the movement from the base of your spine, allowing each vertebra to stack on top of the next.
   - Imagine pulling your belly button towards your spine to support the movement.

- Keep your shoulders relaxed and your chest lifted as you return to an upright position.

5. Repeat:
  - Repeat the forward bend and return to start for a series of repetitions, focusing on smooth, controlled movements and coordinated breathing.
  - Aim to maintain proper alignment and form throughout the exercise, avoiding any strain or discomfort.
  - Start with a small range of motion and gradually increase as your flexibility improves.

6. Variations:
  - To increase the challenge, you can add resistance by placing a resistance band around your feet and holding the ends with your hands.
  - You can also perform the seated spine stretch with your legs slightly wider apart or with a slight external rotation of the hips to target different muscles of the spine and hips.

7. Cool Down:

- After completing the desired number of repetitions, take a moment to sit tall and breathe deeply, allowing your body to relax and release any tension.

- You can follow up with gentle stretches or relaxation exercises to further unwind and restore your body.

Incorporating this exercise into your Pilates routine can help improve spinal flexibility, posture, and overall mobility.

## C. Leg Swings:

Leg swings are dynamic stretching exercises that help to improve hip mobility and flexibility. Here are the steps to perform leg swings:

1. Find a Support: Stand next to a wall, sturdy piece of furniture, or any stable surface that you can hold onto for balance. This support will help you maintain your balance throughout the exercise.

2. Stand Tall: Stand up straight with your feet hip-width apart and your core engaged to maintain stability.

3. Hold onto Support: Hold onto the support with one hand for balance. Keep your shoulders relaxed and your gaze forward.

4. Swing Leg Forward: Shift your weight onto one leg while keeping the other leg relaxed. Swing the relaxed leg forward in a controlled motion, aiming to reach a comfortable range of motion without forcing it.

5. Swing Leg Backward: After completing the forward swing, allow the leg to swing backward, again in a controlled motion. Keep the movement smooth and fluid.

6. Repeat: Perform the leg swings for the desired number of repetitions or for a specific amount of time. Start with a small number of swings and gradually increase as you feel more comfortable and confident with the movement.

7. Switch Sides: Once you have completed the desired number of swings on one leg, switch sides and repeat the exercise with the other leg.

8. Maintain Control: Throughout the exercise, focus on maintaining control and stability. Avoid swinging the leg too forcefully or allowing it to swing beyond a comfortable range of motion.

9. Breathe: Remember to breathe naturally throughout the exercise, inhaling and exhaling in a relaxed manner. Coordinate your breath with the movement to help promote relaxation and fluidity.

10. Cool Down: After completing the leg swings, take a moment to gently shake out your legs and perform any additional stretches or movements to cool down and release any tension in the muscles.

D. Arm swings:

Here are the steps for performing arm swings:

1. Stand with your feet hip-width apart and your arms relaxed by your sides.
2. Engage your core muscles to stabilize your body.
3. Begin swinging your arms forward and backward in a controlled motion.
4. Start with small swings, gradually increasing the range of motion as you warm up.
5. Coordinate your breathing with the movement, inhaling as you swing your arms forward and exhaling as you swing them backward.
6. Keep your shoulders relaxed and avoid locking your elbows.
7. Continue swinging your arms for the desired duration, typically for about 30 seconds to 1 minute.
8. To finish, gradually decrease the intensity of the swings until your arms come to a gentle stop.
9. Take a moment to observe any sensations in your arms and shoulders, and then proceed with your Pilates workout or other exercises.

If you experience any discomfort or pain, reduce the range of motion or stop the exercise altogether.

By incorporating gentle joint movements, breathing techniques, and mobility exercises into their Pilates warm-up routine, seniors can prepare their bodies for the more challenging exercises ahead while reaping the benefits of increased flexibility, improved circulation, and enhanced relaxation. It's important to listen to your body and modify exercises as needed to ensure a safe and enjoyable warm-up experience.

# Chapter 3

# Core Strengthening

Core strengthening is a fundamental aspect of Pilates that help maintain stability, improve posture, and prevent injuries. A strong core provides support for the spine and pelvis, facilitating better balance and mobility in daily activities. In this section, we will explore three core strengthening exercises specifically tailored for you: pelvic tilts, abdominal activations, and modified planks.

# Pelvic Tilts

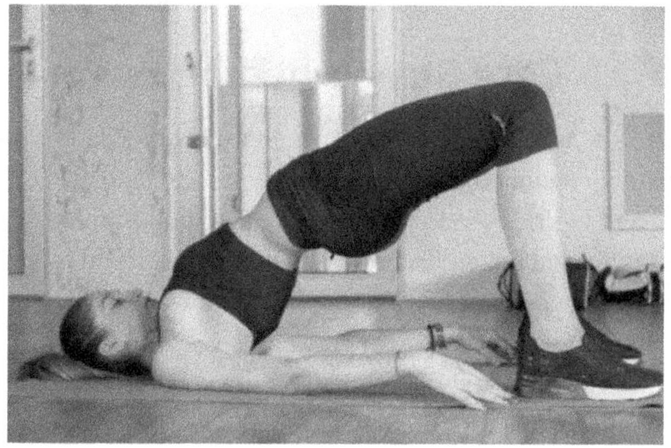

Pelvic tilts are a simple yet effective exercise for strengthening the muscles of the lower back and abdomen. They help to improve pelvic alignment, reduce lower back pain, and enhance core stability. Here's how to perform pelvic tilts:

1. Starting Position: Lie on your back with knees bent and feet flat on the floor, hip-width apart. Place your arms by your sides with palms facing down.

2. Neutral Spine: Begin in a neutral spine position, with a small natural curve in the lower back and the pelvis in a neutral position.

3. Engage Core Muscles: Inhale to prepare, and then exhale as you gently draw your navel toward your spine, engaging the deep abdominal muscles.

4. Tilt Pelvis: Slowly tilt your pelvis backward, flattening the lower back against the mat. You should feel a gentle contraction in the lower abdominals.

5. Hold: Hold the pelvic tilt for a few seconds, maintaining engagement of the core muscles and keeping the pelvis stable.

6. Return to Neutral: Inhale to release the pelvic tilt and return to the neutral spine position.

7. Repeat: Perform 10-15 repetitions, focusing on smooth, controlled movements and maintaining proper alignment throughout.

# Abdominal Activations

Abdominal activations are another effective core strengthening exercise that targets the deep abdominal muscles, including the transverse abdominis. This exercise helps to improve core stability and support spinal alignment. Here's how to perform abdominal activations:

1. Starting Position: Lie on your back with knees bent and feet flat on the floor, hip-width apart. Place your hands on your abdomen, just below the rib cage.

2. Neutral Spine: Begin in a neutral spine position, with a small natural curve in the lower back and the pelvis in a neutral position.

3. Engage Core Muscles: Inhale to prepare, and then exhale as you gently draw your navel toward your spine, contracting the deep abdominal muscles.

4. Hold: Hold the abdominal contraction for 5-10 seconds, maintaining a steady breath and keeping the rest of the body relaxed.

5. Release: Inhale to release the abdominal contraction and return to the neutral spine position.

6. Repeat: Perform 10-15 repetitions, focusing on maintaining proper alignment and control throughout the movement.

## Modified Planks

Modified planks are a modified version of the traditional plank exercise that provides similar benefits for core strength while reducing strain on the wrists and shoulders. This exercise helps seniors develop stability in the core muscles and improve overall body strength. Here's how to perform modified planks:

1. Starting Position: Begin on your hands and knees, with your wrists directly under your shoulders and your knees under your hips. Engage your core muscles to support your spine.

2. Neutral Spine: Maintain a neutral spine position, with a straight line from the top of your head to your tailbone, avoiding any arching or rounding of the back.

3. Engage Core Muscles: Inhale to prepare, and then exhale as you lift your knees off the floor, straightening your legs behind you and coming into a modified plank position.

4. Alignment: Ensure that your body forms a straight line from your head to your heels, with your core muscles engaged and your hips level with your shoulders.

5. Hold: Hold the modified plank position for 10-30 seconds, maintaining steady breathing and focusing on keeping the core muscles activated.

6. Release: Inhale as you lower your knees back to the starting position, returning to the hands and knees position.

7. Repeat: Perform 3-5 repetitions, gradually increasing the duration of the hold as you build strength and endurance.

By incorporating pelvic tilts, abdominal activations, and modified planks into their Pilates routine, seniors can effectively strengthen their core muscles, improve stability, and support spinal alignment. It's important to start slowly and gradually increase the intensity and duration of these exercises as strength and comfort levels improve. Additionally, listen to your body and modify exercises as needed to ensure a safe and enjoyable workout experience.

# Chapter 4

# Enhancing Balance and Stability with Pilates

Balance and stability are vital components of functional movement, particularly as we age. Pilates offers a unique approach to improving balance and stability through a combination of standing poses, proprioception exercises, and coordination drills specifically tailored for seniors. In this section, we will explore these three aspects in detail to help enhance overall stability and confidence in movement.

## Standing Pilates Poses

Standing Pilates poses challenge balance and stability while simultaneously engaging the core muscles and promoting proper alignment. These poses help seniors develop strength, coordination, and proprioception (awareness of body position) in a

weight-bearing position. Here are some standing
Pilates poses suitable for seniors:

A. Tree Pose:

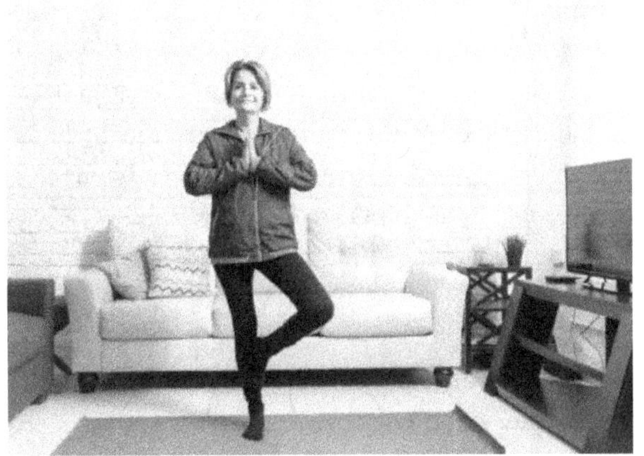

The Tree Pose is a standing yoga posture that
challenges balance, strengthens the legs, and
improves concentration. Here are the steps to
perform the Tree Pose:

1. Starting Position: Begin standing tall with your feet together and arms by your sides. Take a few deep breaths to center yourself and establish a steady foundation.

2. Shift Weight: Shift your weight onto your left foot while keeping the right foot grounded.

3. Lift Leg: Slowly lift your right foot off the ground and place the sole of your right foot against the inner left thigh or calf. Avoid placing the foot directly on the knee to protect the joint. Find a comfortable position where you can maintain balance without straining.

4. Stability: Press the sole of your right foot firmly against the inner left thigh or calf, and engage the muscles of your standing leg for stability. Keep your hips level and facing forward.

5. Hands: Bring your palms together in front of your chest in a prayer position, or extend your arms overhead, reaching toward the sky. Find a gaze point

(or drishti) in front of you to help maintain balance and focus.

6. Balance: Focus on a spot on the floor or wall in front of you to help maintain your balance. Engage your core muscles to support your spine and keep your body steady.

7. Breathing: Take slow, deep breaths as you hold the pose, inhaling through your nose and exhaling through your mouth. Keep your breath steady and relaxed to help calm the mind and deepen your focus.

8. Hold: Hold the Tree Pose for 30 seconds to 1 minute, or as long as feels comfortable for you. If you feel wobbly or unstable, you can use a nearby wall or chair for support until you feel more confident in the pose.

9. Release: Gently lower your right foot back to the ground and return to the starting position with both feet together. Take a moment to notice how you feel after the pose, and then repeat on the other side by

shifting your weight onto your right foot and lifting your left foot into the Tree Pose.

10. Symmetry: Remember to practice the Tree Pose on both sides to maintain balance and symmetry in the body.

The Tree Pose can be modified to suit different levels of flexibility and balance. Beginners may find it helpful to start with the foot placed against the ankle or calf for added stability, gradually working their way up to the inner thigh as they gain strength and confidence. With regular practice, the Tree Pose can help you improve balance, strengthen the legs, and cultivate a sense of calm and focus.

B. Warrior II Pose:

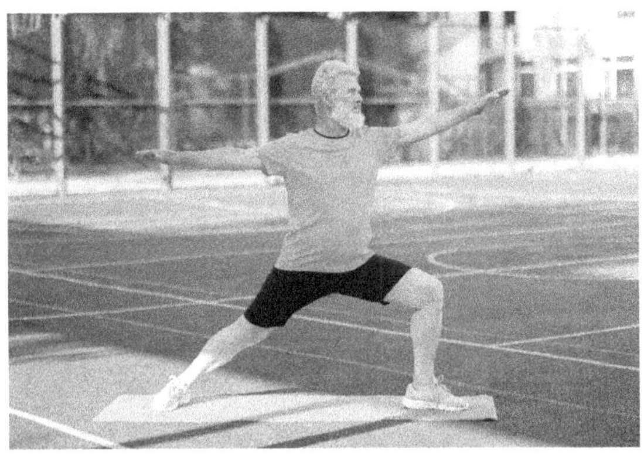

 Warrior II Pose, also known as Virabhadrasana II in Sanskrit, is a foundational standing yoga pose that strengthens the legs, opens the hips, and improves balance and stability. Here are the steps to perform Warrior II Pose:

1. Starting Position: Begin standing at the top of your mat with feet hip-width apart and arms by your sides (Mountain Pose or Tadasana).

2. Step Back: Take a big step back with your left foot, about 3-4 feet behind you. Align the left heel with the arch of your right foot, ensuring that your feet are approximately heel to heel or slightly wider.

3. Open the Hips: Rotate your left hip and foot outward, so they are facing the left side of the mat. Keep your right foot pointing forward.

4. Bend the Front Knee: Bend your right knee, ensuring that it is directly over your right ankle. Aim to create a 90-degree angle with your right thigh parallel to the floor. Adjust the stance of your feet if necessary to achieve proper alignment.

5. Extend the Arms: Extend your arms out to the sides at shoulder height, palms facing down. Your arms should be parallel to the floor, forming a straight line with your shoulders.

6. Gaze: Turn your head to gaze over your right fingertips, keeping your neck long and relaxed. Your gaze should be focused past your front fingertips.

7. Engage the Core: Draw your navel toward your spine to engage the core muscles and stabilize your torso.

8. Square the Hips and Shoulders: Keep your hips and shoulders squared toward the side of the mat, avoiding any twisting or tilting of the torso.

9. Relax the Shoulders: Soften your shoulders away from your ears and broaden across the collarbones.

10. Breathe: Take slow, deep breaths as you hold the pose, maintaining a steady and even rhythm.

11. Hold the Pose: Hold Warrior II Pose for 30 seconds to 1 minute, or longer if comfortable, focusing on your breath and maintaining stability and strength in the legs.

12. Release: To release the pose, straighten your right leg and step your feet back together at the top of the mat. Repeat the pose on the opposite side, stepping the left foot back and bending the left knee. Warrior II Pose is an empowering and grounding posture that builds strength, endurance, and focus. It is often incorporated into yoga sequences and can be practiced as a standalone pose to improve lower body strength and flexibility. As with any yoga pose,

listen to your body, modify as needed, and avoid any discomfort or strain.

C. Chair Pose:

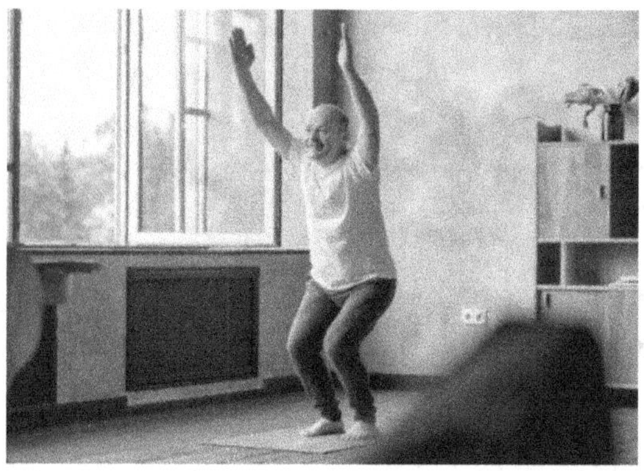

 Chair Pose, also known as Utkatasana in Sanskrit, is a standing yoga posture that strengthens the legs, core, and back while improving balance and focus. Here are the steps to perform Chair Pose:

1. Starting Position: Begin by standing tall with your feet together, arms by your sides, and shoulders relaxed.

2. Mountain Pose (Tadasana): Engage your core muscles and distribute your weight evenly across both feet. Ground down through the four corners of your feet – the big toe mound, pinky toe mound, inner heel, and outer heel – to create a stable foundation.

3. Inhale and Raise Arms: Inhale deeply as you reach your arms overhead, palms facing each other, and fingers spread wide. Lengthen through your spine and keep your shoulders relaxed away from your ears.

4. Exhale and Bend Knees: As you exhale, begin to bend your knees as if sitting back into an imaginary chair. Keep your knees in line with your ankles and your thighs parallel to the floor. Focus on keeping your weight in your heels to activate the muscles in your glutes and hamstrings.

5. Engage Core: Engage your core muscles by drawing your navel toward your spine. This helps to stabilize your torso and protect your lower back.

6. Alignment: Ensure that your knees are aligned with your second toes and avoid letting your knees collapse inward. Keep your chest lifted and your spine long, avoiding rounding or arching in the back.

7. Gaze Forward: Maintain a steady gaze forward, keeping your neck in line with your spine. Relax your facial muscles and breathe deeply as you hold the pose.

8. Hold the Pose: Hold Chair Pose for 30 seconds to 1 minute, or as long as you feel comfortable. Focus on maintaining proper alignment and deepening your breath to help sustain the pose.

9. Release: To release the pose, exhale as you straighten your legs and lower your arms back down by your sides. Stand tall in Mountain Pose for a few breaths to reset before moving on to the next pose.

Tips:
- If you have tight shoulders or find it challenging to raise your arms overhead, you can keep your hands

on your hips or bring them into a prayer position at
your chest.
- If you have knee issues or difficulty balancing, you
can practice Chair Pose against a wall for added
support or reduce the depth of the squat by bending
your knees less.
- Focus on maintaining a steady breath throughout
the pose, inhaling deeply through your nose and
exhaling fully through your mouth.
- As you become more comfortable with Chair Pose,
you can explore variations such as twisting the torso
or lifting onto the balls of your feet for an additional
challenge.

D. Single Leg Balance:

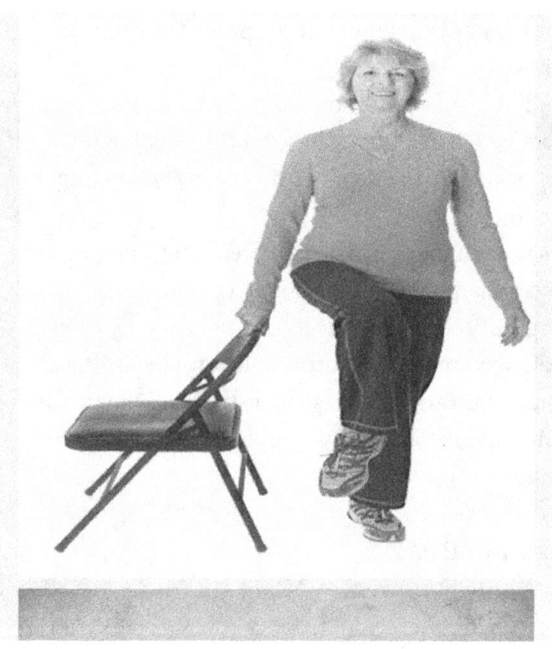

Single leg balance is a fundamental exercise for improving balance, stability, and proprioception. It helps strengthen the muscles of the lower body, including the ankles, knees, and hips, while also engaging the core for stability. Here are the steps to perform single leg balance:

1. Starting Position: Begin by standing tall with your feet hip-width apart and your arms relaxed by your sides.

2. Engage Core Muscles: Activate your core muscles by gently drawing your navel toward your spine. This helps stabilize your pelvis and spine throughout the exercise.

3. Shift Weight: Transfer your weight onto one foot while lifting the opposite foot slightly off the ground. You can either keep the lifted foot hovering just above the floor or place the toes lightly on the ground for additional support.

4. Find Balance: Focus your gaze on a fixed point in front of you to help maintain balance. Avoid looking down at your feet, as this can disrupt your balance.

5. Stabilize: Once you've found your balance on one leg, focus on keeping your standing leg stable and steady. Imagine rooting down through the foot into the ground to create a strong foundation.

6. Alignment: Ensure proper alignment by keeping your hips level and avoiding any tilting or leaning to one side. Your shoulders should also remain square and relaxed.

7. Hold: Hold the single leg balance for 10-30 seconds, or as long as you can maintain proper form without wobbling excessively.

8. Switch Sides: Slowly lower the lifted foot back to the ground and switch to the opposite leg. Repeat the same steps on the other side.

9. Progression: As you become more comfortable with single leg balance, you can challenge yourself by closing your eyes, extending your arms out to the sides or overhead, or adding small movements such as lifting the knee higher or rotating the leg outward.

10. Breathing: Remember to breathe deeply and evenly throughout the exercise. Inhale through your nose to prepare, and exhale through your mouth as you find your balance and hold the position.

11. Repetition: Aim to perform 3-5 repetitions on each leg, gradually increasing the duration of each hold as your balance improves.

12. Cool Down: After completing the single leg balance exercise on both sides, take a moment to stand with both feet planted firmly on the ground and relax your muscles. Shake out any tension and take a few deep breaths before moving on to the next exercise or activity.

Incorporating single leg balance into your regular workout routine can help improve your balance, stability, and overall lower body strength. Start with shorter holds and gradually work your way up to longer durations as you build confidence and stability.

## Proprioception Exercises

Proprioception exercises focus on improving awareness of body position and movement, which is essential for maintaining balance and stability. These exercises challenge the sensory feedback system and help individuals develop better coordination and control. Here are some proprioception exercises suitable for you:

1. Tandem Stance: Stand with one foot directly in front of the other, heel to toe, like walking on a tightrope. Keep your arms by your sides or place your hands on your hips for support. Hold the stance for 30 seconds to 1 minute, then switch sides.

2. Eyes Closed Balance: Stand tall with feet hip-width apart and arms by your sides. Close your eyes and focus on maintaining your balance without visual input. Engage your core muscles and keep your body centered. Hold the pose for 30 seconds to 1 minute, then open your eyes.

3. Dynamic Balance: Stand on one leg and perform small movements with the other leg, such as swinging it forward and backward or circling it in the air. Focus on maintaining your balance on the standing leg while performing the movements. Repeat for 10-15 repetitions, then switch sides.

# Coordination Drills

Coordination drills involve integrating movement patterns from different parts of the body to improve overall coordination and motor control. These drills challenge seniors to synchronize movements and enhance their ability to perform complex tasks with precision and efficiency. Here are some coordination drills suitable for you:

1. Arm and Leg Raises: Stand tall with feet hip-width apart and arms by your sides. Simultaneously raise one arm overhead and lift the opposite leg off the floor, balancing on the standing leg. Lower the arm and leg back to the starting position, then repeat on the other side. Alternate sides for 10-15 repetitions.

2. Cross-Crawl Exercise: Stand tall with feet hip-width apart and arms extended out to the sides at shoulder height. Simultaneously lift one knee toward the opposite elbow, twisting the torso slightly.

Return to the starting position and repeat on the other side. Continue alternating sides for 10-15 repetitions.

3. Marching in Place with Arm Circles: Stand tall with feet hip-width apart and arms by your sides. Lift one knee toward your chest while simultaneously circling the arms forward. Lower the knee and arms back to the starting position, then repeat on the other side. Continue alternating sides for 10-15 repetitions.

 It's important to start slowly and gradually increase the intensity and complexity of these exercises as strength and confidence levels improve. Additionally, seniors should listen to their bodies and modify exercises as needed to ensure a safe and enjoyable workout experience.

# Chapter 5

# Flexibility Training for Seniors in Pilates

Flexibility is a key component of physical fitness that tends to decline with age, leading to stiffness, reduced range of motion, and increased risk of injury. Flexibility training in Pilates focuses on improving the suppleness of muscles and joints, promoting mobility, and enhancing overall functional movement. In this section, we will explore three aspects of flexibility training specifically tailored for seniors in Pilates: gentle stretching routines, range of motion exercises, and the numerous benefits of flexibility for seniors.

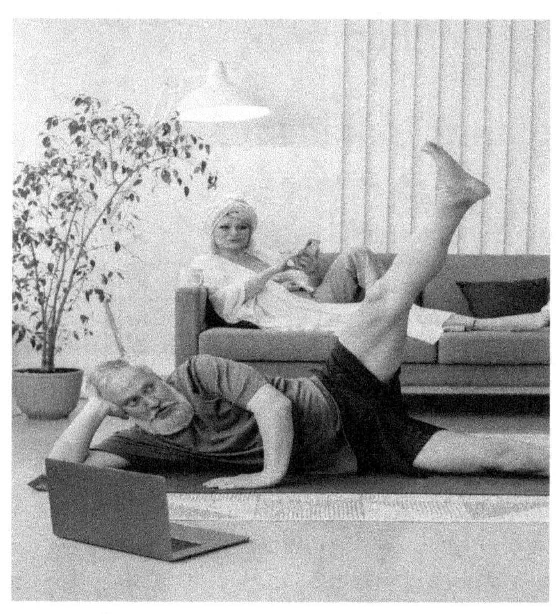

## Gentle Stretching Routines

Gentle stretching routines in Pilates help seniors increase flexibility and release tension in tight muscles, promoting relaxation and a sense of well-being. These stretching exercises are performed with slow, controlled movements and an emphasis on breath awareness. Here are some examples of gentle stretching routines for seniors:

1. Neck Stretch: Sit or stand tall with your shoulders relaxed. Gently tilt your head to one side, bringing your ear toward your shoulder until you feel a stretch along the side of your neck. Hold for 15-30 seconds, then switch sides.

2. Shoulder Stretch: Bring one arm across your body at shoulder height and use the opposite hand to gently press the arm closer to your chest until you feel a stretch in the shoulder and upper back. Hold for 15-30 seconds, then switch sides.

3. Spinal Twist: Sit on the floor with your legs extended in front of you. Bend one knee and place the foot flat on the floor on the outside of the opposite knee. Place the opposite hand on the bent knee and gently twist your torso toward the bent knee, reaching the opposite arm behind you for support. Hold for 15-30 seconds, then switch sides.

4. Hamstring Stretch: Sit on the floor with one leg extended and the other leg bent, foot resting against the inner thigh of the extended leg. Lean forward from the hips, reaching toward the toes of the extended leg until you feel a stretch in the back of the thigh. Hold for 15-30 seconds, then switch legs.

5. Hip Flexor Stretch: Kneel on one knee with the opposite foot flat on the floor in front of you. Press your hips forward slightly until you feel a stretch in the front of the hip of the kneeling leg. Hold for 15-30 seconds, then switch sides.

## Range of Motion Exercises

Range of motion exercises in Pilates help seniors maintain and improve joint mobility, allowing for smoother, more fluid movement in daily activities. These exercises focus on moving joints through their full range of motion in a controlled manner. Here are some examples of range of motion exercises for seniors:

1. Arm Circles: Stand tall with arms extended out to the sides at shoulder height. Circle the arms forward in small, controlled motions, gradually increasing the size of the circles. After several repetitions, reverse the direction of the circles.

2. Leg Swings: Stand next to a wall or sturdy support for balance. Swing one leg forward and backward in a controlled motion, gradually increasing the range of motion with each swing. Repeat on the other leg.

3. Ankle Circles: Sit or stand with feet flat on the floor. Lift one foot off the ground and rotate the ankle in circular motions, first clockwise and then counterclockwise. Repeat on the other foot.

4. Spinal Flexion and Extension: Sit tall on a chair with feet flat on the floor. Inhale as you arch your spine, lifting your chest and looking up toward the ceiling. Exhale as you round your spine, tucking your chin toward your chest. Repeat several times, moving with your breath.

# Flexibility Benefits for Seniors

Flexibility training offers numerous benefits, enhancing both physical and mental well-being. Here are some of the key benefits of flexibility training:

1. Improved Range of Motion: Regular stretching and range of motion exercises help seniors maintain and improve flexibility, allowing for greater freedom of movement in daily activities such as bending, reaching, and twisting.

2. Reduced Risk of Injury: Flexibility training helps seniors maintain muscle and joint health, reducing the risk of strains, sprains, and other injuries. Increased flexibility also improves balance and stability, further reducing the risk of falls.

3. Pain Relief: Stretching can help alleviate stiffness and discomfort associated with tight muscles and restricted range of motion. Gentle stretching routines can help seniors manage chronic pain conditions such as arthritis and fibromyalgia.

4. Enhanced Posture: Improved flexibility in the muscles and joints can help seniors maintain better posture and alignment, reducing the risk of back pain and other musculoskeletal issues.

5. Stress Reduction: Flexibility training promotes relaxation and stress relief, helping seniors unwind and release tension both physically and mentally. Deep breathing and mindfulness techniques incorporated into stretching routines further enhance the relaxation response.

6. Improved Circulation: Stretching and range of motion exercises promote better blood flow to the muscles and joints, delivering oxygen and nutrients while flushing out toxins and waste products. This can help improve overall circulation and cardiovascular health.

7. Increased Mind-Body Awareness: Flexibility training encourages seniors to tune into their bodies, paying attention to sensations, breath, and movement. This heightened awareness fosters a

deeper mind-body connection, promoting overall
well-being and vitality.

 With consistent practice, you can reap the numerous
benefits of flexibility training and enjoy greater
freedom of movement and vitality as you age.

# Chapter 6

# Strength Training for Seniors in Pilates

Strength training is a crucial component of fitness, especially for seniors, as it helps maintain muscle mass, bone density, and overall physical function. Pilates offers safe and effective ways for to engage in strength training, focusing on low-resistance exercises, modified Pilates with props, and building muscular endurance. In this section, we will delve into each aspect to provide a comprehensive understanding of strength training for seniors in Pilates.

## Low-Resistance Exercises

Low-resistance exercises in Pilates involve using the body's own weight as resistance or incorporating light props such as resistance bands, small weights, or Pilates rings. These exercises help seniors build strength gradually without putting undue stress on the joints or risking injury. Here are some examples of low-resistance exercises for seniors in Pilates:

1. Leg Press: Sit tall on a chair with feet flat on the floor and knees bent. Place a small Pilates ball between your knees and squeeze the ball as you extend your legs, pressing against the resistance. Hold for a few seconds, then release and repeat.

2. Arm Circles with Resistance Band: Stand tall with feet hip-width apart and hold one end of a resistance band in each hand. Extend your arms out to the sides at shoulder height and perform small circles with the arms, engaging the shoulder muscles. Gradually increase the size of the circles for greater resistance.

3. Bridge with Resistance Band: Lie on your back with knees bent and feet flat on the floor. Place a resistance band just above the knees and press the knees outward against the resistance as you lift your hips toward the ceiling into a bridge position. Hold for a few seconds, then lower back down and repeat.

4. Side Leg Lifts with Ankle Weights: Lie on your side with legs stacked and ankles weighted. Lift the top leg upward, engaging the outer thigh muscles, then lower back down with control. Repeat for a set number of repetitions, then switch sides.

## Modified Pilates with Props

Modified Pilates exercises with props offer additional resistance and challenge, helping seniors build strength and stability in a controlled manner. Props such as stability balls, Pilates rings, and foam rollers can be incorporated into traditional Pilates exercises to target specific muscle groups and enhance overall strength. Here are some examples of modified Pilates exercises with props for seniors:

1. Stability Ball Squats: Stand tall with a stability ball placed between your lower back and a wall. Lower into a squat position, keeping your knees aligned with your ankles and pressing against the ball for support. Hold for a few seconds, then rise back up and repeat.

2. Pilates Ring Chest Press: Sit tall on a chair with feet flat on the floor and hold a Pilates ring in front of your chest with elbows bent. Press the ring outward, extending your arms fully while engaging the chest muscles. Hold for a few seconds, then release and repeat.

3. Foam Roller Planks: Place a foam roller under your shins and assume a plank position, with hands shoulder-width apart and shoulders stacked over wrists. Engage your core muscles and hold the plank position for as long as you can maintain proper form, focusing on stability and control.

4. Resistance Band Rows: Sit tall on a chair with feet flat on the floor and loop a resistance band around the bottom of your feet. Hold one end of the band in each hand and perform rows by pulling the band toward your chest, engaging the back muscles. Slowly release and repeat for a set number of repetitions.

Building Muscular Endurance

In addition to building strength, you can benefit from focusing on muscular endurance, which refers to the ability of muscles to perform repetitive contractions over an extended period of time. Pilates offers exercises that target specific muscle groups and challenge endurance while promoting proper alignment and control. Here are some strategies for building muscular endurance through Pilates:

1. High-Repetition Sets: Perform exercises for higher repetitions, aiming for 12-15 repetitions per set to fatigue the muscles and promote endurance.

2. Slow and Controlled Movements: Emphasize slow and controlled movements to engage the muscles more effectively and prolong the time under tension.

3. Pilates Circuit Training: Incorporate a circuit-style workout with multiple exercises targeting different muscle groups. Perform each exercise for a set duration or number of repetitions before moving on

to the next exercise, allowing minimal rest between sets to maintain intensity and challenge endurance.

4. Progressive Overload: Gradually increase the intensity or resistance of exercises over time to continue challenging the muscles and promoting adaptations. This can be achieved by using heavier weights, increasing resistance band tension, or adjusting the difficulty of Pilates exercises.

 With consistent practice and dedication you can reap the numerous benefits of strength training in Pilates, leading to greater independence, vitality, and quality of life.

# Chapter 7

# Enhancing Posture with Pilates for Seniors

Maintaining good posture is essential to prevent discomfort, reduce the risk of injury, and promote overall well-being. Pilates offers a variety of exercises and techniques specifically designed to improve posture by strengthening core muscles, stabilizing the spine, and promoting proper alignment. Additionally, incorporating ergonomic tips into daily life can further support healthy posture habits. In this section, we will explore Pilates exercises for better posture, ergonomic tips for daily life, and spine-stabilizing exercises to help achieve and maintain optimal posture.

# Pilates Exercises for Better Posture

Pilates is renowned for its focus on core strength, alignment, and body awareness, making it an ideal practice for improving posture. Here are some Pilates exercises specifically targeted at enhancing posture:

1. Pelvic Tilts: Lie on your back with knees bent and feet flat on the floor. Inhale to prepare, then exhale as you tilt your pelvis backward, flattening your lower back against the mat. Hold for a moment, then inhale to return to neutral. This exercise strengthens the core and encourages proper pelvic alignment.

2. Chest Opener: Sit tall with legs extended in front of you and a small Pilates ball or cushion between your hands. Inhale as you reach your arms overhead, opening your chest and lifting your gaze. Exhale as you lower your arms, squeezing the ball between your palms. This exercise helps counteract rounded shoulders and encourages thoracic extension.

3. Scapular Retraction: Stand tall with arms extended out to the sides at shoulder height. Inhale to prepare, then exhale as you draw your shoulder blades together, squeezing them gently. Hold for a moment, then inhale to release. This exercise strengthens the muscles between the shoulder blades and promotes proper shoulder alignment.

4. Spine Stretch Forward: Sit tall with legs extended in front of you, feet flexed. Inhale to lengthen your spine, then exhale as you hinge forward from the hips, reaching your hands toward your feet. Keep your back flat and avoid rounding the spine. This exercise stretches the hamstrings and promotes spinal articulation.

## Ergonomic Tips for Daily Life

In addition to Pilates exercises, incorporating ergonomic principles into daily activities can help you maintain good posture and reduce strain on the body. Here are some ergonomic tips to improve posture in daily life:

1. Sit and Stand Tall: Whether sitting or standing, maintain a neutral spine with shoulders relaxed and aligned over the hips. Avoid slouching or arching the back, and engage core muscles to support proper posture.

2. Use Supportive Furniture: Choose chairs and mattresses that provide adequate support for the spine and promote good posture. Use cushions or lumbar rolls if additional support is needed to maintain proper spinal alignment.

3. Adjust Workspace Setup: Ensure that computer screens are at eye level, keyboards are positioned at elbow height, and chairs provide proper lumbar support. Take regular breaks to stand up, stretch, and move around to prevent stiffness and promote circulation.

4. Lift Safely: When lifting objects, bend at the knees and hips rather than the waist, and keep the spine neutral. Use your leg muscles to lift, and avoid twisting or jerking movements that can strain the back.

# Spine-Stabilizing Exercises

Stabilizing the spine is crucial for maintaining good posture and preventing injuries. Pilates offers a variety of exercises that target the muscles supporting the spine, helping to improve stability and reduce the risk of back pain. Here are some spine-stabilizing exercises:

1. Bird Dog: Begin on hands and knees with wrists under shoulders and knees under hips. Inhale to prepare, then exhale as you extend one arm forward and the opposite leg backward, maintaining a flat back and engaging core muscles. Hold for a moment, then return to the starting position and switch sides. This exercise strengthens the muscles of the core and stabilizes the spine.

2. Plank:

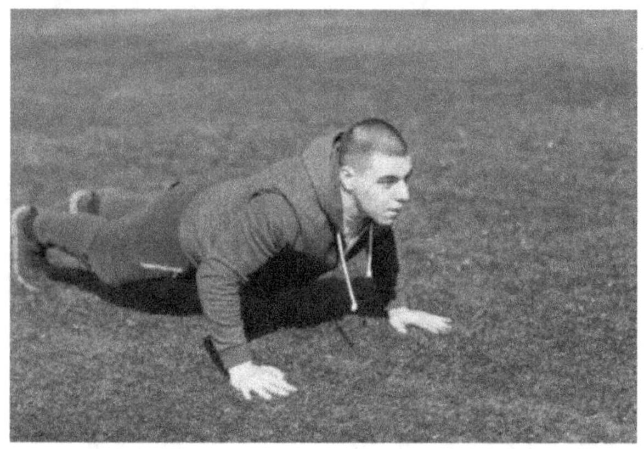

Start in a push-up position with hands under shoulders and body in a straight line from head to heels. Engage core muscles and hold the position for as long as you can maintain proper form, focusing on stabilizing the spine and avoiding sagging or arching. This exercise strengthens the entire core and promotes spinal alignment.

3. Side Plank: Lie on one side with legs stacked and elbow directly under shoulder. Lift your hips off the mat, creating a straight line from head to heels, and engage core muscles to stabilize the spine. Hold for

as long as you can maintain proper form, then lower back down and switch sides. This exercise targets the muscles of the side body and promotes lateral stability of the spine.

Incorporating Pilates exercises for better posture, ergonomic tips for daily life, and spine-stabilizing exercises into a regular routine can help seniors maintain optimal posture, reduce discomfort, and support overall spinal health.

# Chapter 8

# Enhancing Well-being: Relaxation, Mindfulness, and Stress Reduction with Pilates

In the realm of holistic health and fitness, relaxation, mindfulness, and stress reduction play pivotal roles in achieving overall well-being. For seniors embarking on a Pilates journey, integrating these elements into their practice is not just beneficial but also essential for maximizing the benefits of their workouts. In this chapter, we will delve into various relaxation techniques, explore the significance of mindful breathing, and uncover stress reduction exercises through Pilates tailored specifically for seniors.

Relaxation Techniques

1. Progressive Muscle Relaxation (PMR): PMR involves systematically tensing and relaxing different muscle groups to alleviate physical tension and induce a state of deep relaxation. Seniors can incorporate PMR into their Pilates routine by consciously engaging and then releasing muscle groups during specific exercises. This technique enhances body awareness and promotes relaxation, making it an ideal complement to Pilates movements.

2. Guided Imagery: Guided imagery taps into the power of visualization to promote relaxation and reduce stress. During Pilates sessions, instructors can guide seniors through visualizations of tranquil settings, such as a peaceful beach or a serene garden. By immersing themselves in these mental images, seniors can create a sense of calm and well-being, enhancing the overall Pilates experience.

3. Breathing Exercises: Deep breathing techniques are fundamental to relaxation and mindfulness practices. Seniors can incorporate mindful breathing

into their Pilates routine by focusing on deep, diaphragmatic breaths that synchronize with movement. Encouraging seniors to inhale deeply through the nose, allowing the abdomen to expand, and exhale slowly through the mouth fosters relaxation, reduces stress, and enhances concentration during Pilates exercises.

## Mindful Breathing

Mindful breathing is a cornerstone of Pilates practice, facilitating a deeper connection between the mind and body. For seniors, mindful breathing offers a pathway to greater self-awareness, relaxation, and mental clarity. Here are some strategies for integrating mindful breathing into Pilates sessions:

- Breath Awareness: Encourage seniors to pay attention to the natural rhythm of their breath as they move through Pilates exercises. By cultivating awareness of the breath, seniors can enhance their focus, reduce distractions, and deepen their connection to the present moment.

- Breath Synchronization: Guide seniors to synchronize their breath with movement during Pilates exercises. Inhaling during the preparatory phase of an exercise and exhaling during the execution phase fosters smooth, controlled movement and promotes relaxation.

- Focused Attention: Remind seniors to maintain focused attention on their breath throughout the entirety of their Pilates practice. When distractions arise or the mind wanders, encourage seniors to gently redirect their focus back to the breath, fostering a sense of mindfulness and presence.

## Stress Reduction Exercises through Pilates

Pilates offers a multitude of stress reduction exercises that cater to seniors' unique needs and abilities. By incorporating mindful movement, controlled breathing, and relaxation techniques,

Pilates can serve as a powerful tool for managing stress and promoting overall well-being. Here are some stress reduction exercises tailored for seniors:

1. Gentle Stretching: Pilates exercises that focus on gentle stretching and lengthening of the muscles can help seniors release tension and reduce stress. Movements such as the Cat-Cow stretch, Spine Stretch Forward, and Swan Dive encourage flexibility, mobility, and relaxation throughout the body.

2. Breath-Centered Movements: Many Pilates exercises emphasize the importance of coordinating movement with breath, promoting a sense of calm and relaxation. Seniors can engage in breath-centered movements such as the Hundred, Roll-Up, and Single Leg Stretch to cultivate mindfulness, reduce stress, and enhance overall well-being.

3. Mindful Movement Sequences: Pilates sequences that flow smoothly from one movement to the next can promote relaxation and mental clarity. Seniors

can participate in mindful movement sequences such as the Classical Pilates Mat series or a gentle Pilates flow to synchronize breath with movement, reduce stress, and improve overall mood and outlook.

In conclusion, relaxation, mindfulness, and stress reduction are integral components of a Pilates practice tailored for seniors. By incorporating relaxation techniques, mindful breathing, and stress reduction exercises into their Pilates routine, seniors can experience profound physical, mental, and emotional benefits. With regular practice and a commitment to self-care, Pilates can become not only a form of exercise but also a pathway to greater well-being and vitality in the senior years.

# Chapter 9

# Progression and Modifications

Progression and modifications are key aspects of a successful Pilates practice. As individuals age, their bodies may have different needs and abilities, making it essential to tailor exercises to accommodate these changes. In this chapter, we will explore how individuals can gradually advance in their Pilates exercises, adapt movements to meet their individual needs, and effectively monitor their progress along the way.

## Gradual Advancement in Exercises

Building Strength and Endurance: Approach Pilates with a focus on gradual progression, gradually increasing the intensity and complexity of the exercises over time. By starting with foundational movements and gradually incorporating more challenging variations, you can build strength, endurance, and confidence in your Pilates practice.

Mindful Progression: It's important to listen to your body and progress at a pace that feels comfortable and sustainable. You're encouraged to pay attention to how your bodies respond to each exercise and to make adjustments accordingly. Progression should be gradual and mindful, ensure that you feel challenged but not overwhelmed by the Pilates practice.

Variety and Adaptation: Introducing variety into Pilates sessions can help you continue to progress and avoid plateaus in your fitness journey. Incorporating different props, equipment, and movement variations can challenge the body in new ways, promoting continued growth and improvement over time.

## Adapting Pilates Moves for Individual Needs

Customizing Exercises: Pilates exercises can be easily adapted to accommodate seniors with varying abilities and limitations. You're encouraged to work with a qualified Pilates instructor who can tailor exercises to your individual needs, taking into account any physical limitations, injuries, or health concerns.

Modifying for Mobility: People with limited mobility can benefit from modifications that make Pilates exercises more accessible and comfortable. This may involve using props such as blocks, straps, or resistance bands to support and assist with movements, or modifying exercises to be performed in a seated or reclined position.

Focus on Alignment and Stability:  By focusing on alignment cues and engaging the core muscles, seniors can improve posture, balance, and overall body awareness, reducing the risk of injury and enhancing the effectiveness of their workouts.

# Monitoring Progress

Setting Goals: Set specific, achievable goals , whether it's improving flexibility, increasing strength, or reducing pain and discomfort. Setting clear goals provides you with a sense of direction and motivation, that will help you stay focused and committed to your practice.

Tracking Progress: Track your progress by keeping a Pilates journal or log, recording details such as the exercises performed, the duration of each session, and any observations or insights gained during practice. Monitoring progress allows you to track improvements over time and make adjustments as needed to continue progressing toward their goals.

Listening to the Body: Above all, listen to your body and honor your physical limitations. Pilates is a practice of self-awareness and self-care, you should feel empowered to modify exercises or take breaks as needed to ensure safety and well-being during practice.

By gradually advancing in exercises, adapting movements to meet individual needs, and effectively monitoring progress, you can enjoy a safe, effective, and rewarding Pilates experience that supports their overall health and well-being for years to come.

# Chapter 10

# Frequently Asked Questions About Pilates

Pilates is a popular form of exercise among seniors due to its gentle yet effective approach to improving strength, flexibility, and overall well-being. However people may have questions or concerns about starting or maintaining a Pilates practice. In this chapter, we will address some common questions and provide tips for consistency in Pilates practice.

## Addressing Common Concerns

1. Is Pilates Safe for Seniors?
   - Yes, Pilates is generally safe for seniors, but it's essential to consult with a healthcare provider before starting any new exercise program, especially if you have pre-existing health conditions or physical limitations. A qualified Pilates instructor can also

provide modifications to ensure exercises are safe and appropriate for your individual needs.

2. Will Pilates Help with Balance and Fall Prevention?
   - Yes, Pilates can improve balance, stability, and coordination, which are crucial for fall prevention in seniors. Pilates exercises focus on strengthening the core muscles, improving posture, and enhancing body awareness, all of which contribute to better balance and reduced risk of falls.

3. Can Pilates Help with Joint Pain and Arthritis?
   - Yes, Pilates can be beneficial for seniors with joint pain and arthritis. The low-impact nature of Pilates exercises, combined with its focus on gentle, controlled movements, can help alleviate pain, improve flexibility, and increase joint mobility. However, it's essential to communicate any discomfort or limitations to your instructor to ensure exercises are adapted accordingly.

4. Do I Need Special Equipment for Pilates?

- While Pilates can be performed using specialized equipment such as reformers, Cadillac, or chairs, it can also be done using just a mat. Many Pilates exercises can be adapted for mat-based practice, making it accessible and convenient for seniors to do at home or in a group class setting.

## Tips for Consistency

1. Set Realistic Goals: Define specific, achievable goals for your Pilates practice, such as improving flexibility, increasing strength, or reducing stress. Setting realistic goals helps maintain motivation and focus, making it easier to stay consistent with your practice.

2. Find a Supportive Community: Joining a Pilates class or group can provide accountability, encouragement, and camaraderie, making it more likely for you to stick to your practice. Connecting with others who share similar goals and interests can help you stay motivated and inspired on your Pilates journey.

3. Incorporate Pilates into Your Routine: Make Pilates a regular part of your weekly routine by scheduling sessions at a consistent time and day. Whether it's first thing in the morning, during your lunch break, or in the evening before bed, finding a time that works for you and sticking to it can help establish a consistent practice habit.

4. Listen to Your Body: Pay attention to how your body feels during and after Pilates sessions, and adjust your practice accordingly. If you're feeling fatigued or experiencing discomfort, it's okay to take a break or modify exercises to suit your needs. Consistency is about finding a balance between challenging yourself and respecting your body's limits.

5. Celebrate Progress: Celebrate your achievements and milestones along the way, no matter how small they may seem. Whether it's mastering a new exercise, increasing flexibility, or feeling more energized and confident, acknowledging your

progress can boost motivation and reinforce your
commitment to consistent Pilates practice.

Pilates offers numerous benefits , but it's essential to
address common concerns and establish strategies
for consistency to reap the full rewards of this
transformative practice.

# Conclusion

# Embracing the Benefits of Pilates

As we come to the end of this journey through Pilates for seniors, it's essential to reflect on the numerous benefits of this transformative practice and to offer encouragement for embracing a lifelong Pilates journey. From improved strength and flexibility to enhanced balance and mental well-being, Pilates offers a wealth of advantages for seniors seeking to enhance their quality of life and maintain their vitality as they age.

## Recap of Benefits

Throughout this book, we've explored the myriad benefits of Pilates for seniors, including:

- Improved Strength and Flexibility: Pilates exercises target the core muscles and promote functional strength and flexibility, which are essential for maintaining mobility and independence as we age.

- Enhanced Balance and Coordination: Pilates emphasizes proper alignment and body awareness, helping seniors improve balance, stability, and coordination, reducing the risk of falls and injury.

- Reduced Joint Pain and Arthritis: The gentle, low-impact nature of Pilates exercises can help alleviate joint pain and stiffness associated with conditions such as arthritis, promoting greater comfort and mobility.

- Stress Reduction and Mental Well-being: Pilates incorporates mindful breathing and relaxation techniques that promote stress reduction, improved mood, and mental clarity, enhancing overall well-being and quality of life.

## Encouragement for a Lifelong Pilates Practice

As you embark on your Pilates journey, remember that consistency and dedication are key to reaping the full benefits of this practice. Whether you're new to Pilates or a seasoned practitioner, there's always room for growth and improvement. Embrace the process, be patient with yourself, and celebrate your progress along the way.

Pilates is not just a form of exercise; it's a way of life—a practice that can enrich your physical, mental, and emotional well-being for years to come. As you continue on your Pilates journey, may you find joy, vitality, and a renewed sense of vitality with each movement and breath.

To get started with Pilates, here are some recommended equipment:

1. Pilates Mat: A high-quality Pilates mat provides cushioning and support during floor exercises and

helps maintain proper alignment throughout your practice.

2. Resistance Bands: Resistance bands are versatile tools that can be used to add resistance and intensity to Pilates exercises, helping build strength and improve muscle tone.

3. Pilates Ring (Magic Circle): A Pilates ring is a small, lightweight resistance tool that can be used to target specific muscle groups and add variety to your Pilates routine.

4. Stability Ball: A stability ball can be used to challenge balance, stability, and core strength during Pilates exercises, making them more dynamic and engaging.

5. Foam Roller: A foam roller can be used for self-massage and myofascial release, helping relieve muscle tension and improve flexibility, making it an excellent addition to your Pilates practice.

By investing in the right equipment and finding online classes that suit your needs and preferences, you can enjoy the benefits of Pilates from the comfort of your own home, anytime and anywhere.

Pilates offer a holistic approach to health and fitness, promoting strength, flexibility, balance, and mental well-being. By embracing the benefits of Pilates and incorporating it into your daily routine, you can enjoy a vibrant and active lifestyle well into your golden years. So, roll out your mat, take a deep breath, and embark on your Pilates journey with confidence and enthusiasm. Your body, mind, and spirit will thank you for it.